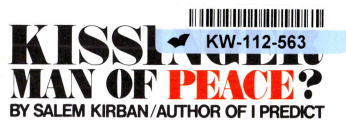

KISSINGER
MAN OF PEACE?

BY SALEM KIRBAN/AUTHOR OF I PREDICT

ACKNOWLEDGMENTS

To **Dr. Gary G. Cohen,** Professor of Greek and New Testament at Biblical School of Theology, Hatfield, Pa., who carefully checked the final manuscript.

To **Robert Krauss,** artist, who designed the front cover.

To **Doreen Frick,** who carefully proofread the text.

Published by SALEM KIRBAN, Inc., Kent Road, Huntingdon Valley, Penna., 19006. Copyright © 1974 by Salem Kirban. Printed in the United States of America. All rights reserved, including the right to reproduce this book or portions thereof in any form.

Library of Congress Catalog Card No. 74-79613
ISBN 0-912582-18-9

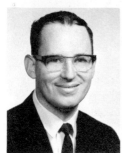

DEDICATION
To **DR. GARY G. COHEN**

I am indebted to Dr. Cohen for his counsel in the preparation of my books. Such a friend is invaluable! Dr. Cohen is of Hebrew heritage and I, of Arab heritage. And while the Middle East conflict has pitted Arab against Jew how thrilling to know that "...ye are all one in Christ Jesus." (Galatians 3:28)

THE JERUSALEM POST MAGAZINE

Friday, January 18, 1974

Henry the Peacemaker

WHY I WROTE THIS BOOK

It is a sad bit of irony that man is able to construct a vehicle that can convey him safely on a 500,000-mile trip through space, but unable to design a table that will accommodate him so that he might embark upon a journey to peace!

In the last few years the world has suffered agonizing pains of constant turmoil...from the prolonged Vietnam War, the energy crisis, the Yom Kippur War, kidnappings, riots, and runaway inflation.

Is it no wonder that people worldwide are looking for a Superman. During the Vietnam War...the cream of intelligent leaders of the world were gathered to resolve the conflict. But first, they decided to play a game. Now most people would tire of playing a game after one or two hours. But these grown men played this game for 8 months! The name of the game was "Shall the Table be round...or shall the Table be square?" At that time Henry Kissinger was the chief negotiator for the U.S.

Yet how can anyone believe that man himself can achieve a Heaven here on earth when it took 8 months of argument just to settle the shape of the peace table in Paris...during the course of which some 8000 more U.S. soldiers lost their lives in Vietnam!

In spite of all this, many people believe the world will get better and peace will be achieved. The world is looking for a Magician...a man who can bring peace...particularly in the war-torn Middle East. To some, Henry Alfred Kissinger looms on the horizon as the saviour of mankind. As London *Times* Foreign Editor Louis Heren recently put it: "Much of the world, East as well as West, hankers for Superman. The role was thrust upon him [Henry Kissinger], although presumably he did not have to be persuaded."

So sure are some that this one man can achieve peace that a constitutional amendment has been proposed to allow foreign-born, naturalized U.S. citizens to be President. Kissinger was born in Germany.

But peace will never be achieved by man. But the curtain of tomorrow may soon be lifted to reveal a man whose peace will unleash an avalanche of terror...such as the world has never seen. That's why this book was written!

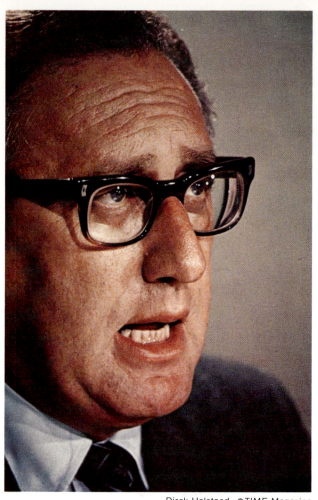

Dirck Halstead ©TIME Magazine

HEINZ ... His Beginning

It was half past six in the evening.

The date was April 20th, 1889.

At that time, a man was born who was to affect drastically the course of history, and whose career was to have a great bearing on the life of a little boy named Heinz, who was to be born May 27th, 1923.

For, by a unique set of circumstances, Adolf Hitler was thrust into power in Germany through some backstair intrigue in 1933. Shortly after that he said, "The extermination of the Jews is not a necessary evil..., it is just necessary!"

Only 10 years earlier, on May 27, 1923, Heinz Alfred Kissinger (who later changed his name to Henry A. Kissinger), was born in Furth, just five miles from Nuremberg.

Heinz Kissinger learned at an early age what it meant to be a Jew...although in later years he said that this experience did not affect him one way or another.

On many occasions he was beaten up by his classmates on his way to school—classmates who were training for Hitler's Youth Movement. Kissinger's father, Louis, was a quiet man who taught in a girl's high school. He and his wife, Paula, had two sons, Heinz, who became Henry, and Walter, who was one year younger.

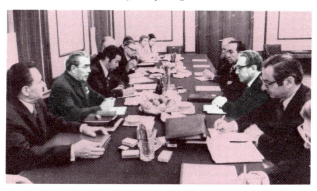

Henry Kissinger Listens as Soviet Communist Party Secretary Leonid Brezhnev speaks. Photo taken during talks at Kremlin, October, 1973.

Shortly after Hitler became Chancellor, the first concentration camps were opened and the threat to the lives of Jews suddenly became a reality.

Hitler's first step was to dismiss all Jews from public employment.

He next confiscated $9 Billion worth of Jewish property, and a general harrassment of the Jews began.

Then, in 1938, he gave orders to destroy every synagogue in Germany. In one month, 35,000 Jews were then put in the concentration camps. A Jewish person could not have more than $2,000, the rest became the property of the state. Finally, Jews were even thrown out of the public schools.

Of his childhood, Henry Kissinger states,

> That part of my childhood is not a key to anything. I was not consciously unhappy. I was not so acutely aware of what was going on. For children, those things are not that serious. It is fashionable now to explain everything psychoanalytically, but let me tell you the political persecutions of my childhood are not what control my life.

Henry Kissinger's friends do not agree with this statement. In fact, twelve of Henry Kissinger's relatives died at the hands of Nazi's before Henry was fourteen years old.

Flight to Freedom

The pressure on the Jews became so great that finally Henry Kissinger's mother and father decided that they would leave Germany for London.

This they did in 1938, and they were among the last of the Jews to be able to escape from Hitler's Germany, for they left just in time.

While in London, an aunt made arrangements for them to leave for New York City.

In New York, Louis Kissinger's wife, Paula, supported the family as a cook for neighbors.

It was impossible for Louis Kissinger to secure a job as a teacher in America, and so he took a job as a clerk—but his heart was always in Germany.

Henry Kissinger attended George Washington High School, and became a straight "A" scholar.

Had not Hitler persecuted the Jews, Henry Kissinger would probably today be a teacher in Germany.

But through this unique set of circumstances, Henry Kissinger was forced out of Germany, to the United States, and through a minor miracle, rose from immigrant status to that of Secretary of State of the United States.

Walter Bernhard Kissinger is Henry's younger brother, and is a quiet millionaire in upstate New York.

Five years after the brothers arrived in America, they were both inducted in the United States Army.

HIS FIRST MARRIAGE

Henry Kissinger was sent to Europe where he was active during the American occupation of Europe. Little is written about Henry Kissinger's ex-wife, Ann Fleischer.

She, too, as Henry, was a refugee. She dated Henry Kissinger for nearly seven years prior to their marriage in 1949. They both had similar jobs, working at night addressing envelopes, and this is where they met.

Ann kept on working to help finance Henry Kissinger's years as a Harvard student.

Apparently the marriage was not a happy one, because of Henry Kissinger's dedication to his work. It has been said that when he would return home at night, he would be so busy anticipating his next day's work, that he would request his wife or anyone else in the house not to talk. Ann Fleischer said that this arrangement added up to a totally, "unhappy marriage."

After fifteen years, the Kissingers' got divorced. They have two children, Elizabeth and David—both teenagers.

His Army Experience

While in the United States Army, Henry Kissinger's first job was as a clerk in a counter-intelligence unit at Camp Gordon, Georgia. This was where German prisoners were kept at the time.

He was soon recognized for his sharp, analytical mind, and was quickly designated to be an interpreter for the 84th division that was sent to Germany. He was noted for his uncanny ability to find his way out of the most difficult situations, and to get stagnant government bureaus moving again.

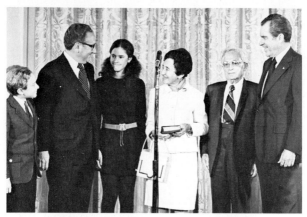

SECRETARY OF STATE KISSINGER WITH HIS SON DAVID, DAUGHTER ELIZABETH, MOTHER PAULA, FATHER LOUIS AND PRESIDENT NIXON.

SPEAK OUT, MR. KISSINGER!

In 1938 Louis Kissinger, a high school administrator in Furth, Germany, took his wife Paula, and their two sons, Henry and Walter, and fled to England to avoid persecution and possible death by Hitler's Nazis. Eleven members of their family stayed behind and eventually lost their lives.

The exodus of the Kissinger family from Hitler Germany was made possible by the vociferous outrage of the British and U.S. governments and the force of public opinion throughout the civilized world.

Last month, Sen. Henry "Scoop" Jackson (D., Wash.) led the move in Congress to prevent granting the most-favored-nation tariff treatment to the Soviet Union so long as that government continued to curb human and emigration rights of its dissenting citizens.

Ironically, one of the men who urged Congress not to link trade with emigration was Henry Kissinger, the new Secretary of State. Kissinger explained that we must not try to change the "domestic structure" of other nations or "we will find ourselves massively involved in every country in the world."

No one wants to antagonize the Soviet Union or revive the days of the Cold War, but the freedom to speak out as human beings, to inveigh openly against the tyrannies and injustices of foreign powers -- that, Mr. Secretary, is what this nation is all about.

Reprinted from PARADE Magazine.

His successes in Germany were so dramatic—even as a young man of 22—that the generals soon were raving to their colleagues about this unusual private.

Soon he was given the job of administering the entire German district of Bergstrasse.

He did such a good job there that he was then given authority to make unlimited arrests of German Nationals.

This authority extended for any legal reason he thought applicable within this district.

His headquarters was a castle in Bergstrasse. Soon he became a sergeant and was transferred to the faculty of the European Command Intelligence School. When his Army tour was ended, the Army hired him to stay on at this same school as a civilian teacher.

But finally he decided that what he really wanted was a college education, so he attended Harvard University, and at last received his Ph.D. degree at that school. Kissinger was to spend several years as an Associate Professor of Government, and finally he became Professor in 1962 at Harvard University.

During Dwight D. Eisenhower's term as President, Kissinger was asked to serve as a foreign policy strategist.

For a brief time, he worked with John F. Kennedy, but became disenchanted with the Kennedy administration, and the "New Frontier."

He then worked briefly for President Lyndon B. Johnson on a project in Vietnam.

One of Henry Kissinger's best loves was that of writing. In 1958, he published a book called, "Nuclear Weapons and Foreign Policy."

This became a best seller.

KISSINGER, Rockefeller and Red China

Henry Kissinger's next job was as Special Studies Director for the Rockefeller foundation. It is interesting to note that back in 1968, Governor Rockefeller was the only real opposition to Richard Nixon at the Republican convention in Miami.

And in one of Rockefeller's press reports—written by

Henry Kissinger—it was suggested that the President of the United States should visit Red China. This was Henry Kissinger's idea, back in 1968.

But it would take several years before this idea would reach fruition.

1968 was the year that several people spent millions of dollars to be elected President. And it was a plume in Rockefeller's cap to be able to have Henry Kissinger on his team.

It is reported that Rockefeller spent $8 million running for this election, while Senator Eugene McCarthy spent $11 million, and Senator Robert Kennedy spent $9 million.

Richard Nixon won the Presidential election and he remembered the effectiveness of Henry Kissinger's work with Nelson Rockefeller.

Because of this, and for other reasons, he sent for Kissinger. A secret meeting was held at the Hotel Pierre in New York. After that meeting, Henry Kissinger became the Assistant to the President for National Security Affairs. The year was 1968. Henry Kissinger had come a long way since his naturalization in 1943. Much of his success he owed to Nelson Rockefeller.

Here was a former brush salesman, who became an Army private, who then served as an interpreter for a General, who then took over a district in Germany...Henry Kissinger ...who was now given his own brigadier general as his personal aide.

Henry Kissinger was to move fast.

In less than a month, he became not only the most powerful figure on foreign policy in this country...but he also became the second most powerful man in the United States government!

The German Trio

Perhaps the most unusual thing about this tie was that Henry Kissinger was to be the most unlikely member of what could be called, "the German trio." The other two members of this trio were H. R. (Bob) Haldeman, whose title was Assistant to the President, and John D. Ehrlichman, whose title was Assistant to the President for Domestic Affairs.

Ehrlichman and Haldeman were classmates at U.C.L.A. They were even Eagle Scouts together, and they attended the Christian Scientist Church together.

It was Henry Kissinger who developed the new National Security Council, and Kissinger's increasing powers and activities were soon to make Secretary of State Rogers simply a figurehead.

It soon became obvious who was the real Secretary of State, and that this man was Henry Kissinger. He quickly held twelve secret meetings with the North Vietnamese officials in Paris. Then President Nixon's trip to China became a reality in February of 1972, also after a series of secret meetings held by Henry Kissinger.

Further, even President Nixon's summit session in Moscow in May of 1972 became a reality only after secret meetings held by Henry Kissinger and the Russians. In crisis after crisis, it was Henry Kissinger's name which always came to the forefront.

In an offhand quip that reveals the demand on this man's time, he was quoted as saying in 1969:

> There cannot be a crisis next week. My schedule's already full.

In 1962, President Nixon wrote in his book "Six Crises," the following very revealing statement:

> **Admitting Red China to the United Nations would be a mockery of the provisions of the charter which limits its membership to 'Peace-loving nations'....**It would give respectability to the Communist regime which would immensely increase its power and prestige in Asia, and probably irreparably weaken the non-Communist governments in that area.

It is singularly important to note that it didn't take long for Henry Kissinger to change the President's mind. The United States' recognition of Red China became a fact in October, 1971.

The Feminine Touch

Along with Henry Kissinger's ability to meet with heads of State, was his ability to secure dates with some of the world's most attractive women.

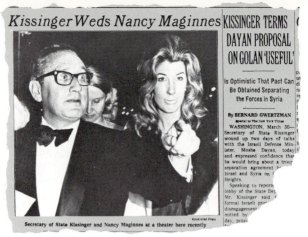

Henry Kissinger with his wife, the former Nancy Maginnes. They were married March 30, 1974 in Alexandria, Virginia.

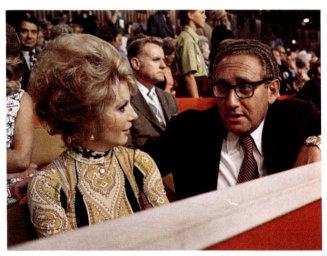

Henry Kissinger with feminine guest at 1972 Miami Republican Convention. On March 30, 1974 he secretly married Nancy Maginnes.

Included in his social itinerary at one time or another were Jill St. John, a movie star; Zsa Zsa Gabor; and Judy Brown, who starred in a Danish film which at least one book referred to as "pornographic."

His other dates included Marlo Thomas, television actress; Angel Tompkins; Barbara Hower; Nancy Maginnes; and CBS News producer, Margaret Osmer.

His Second Marriage

Henry Kissinger, 50, is full of surprises! And he surprised everyone when on Saturday, March 30, 1974 he secretly married his longtime close friend, Nancy Maginnes, 39 in Arlington, Virginia. Nancy is 5 ft. 10 1/2 in., compared with Henry's 5 ft. 8 in. The new Mrs. Kissinger has been described by some as nervous...she smokes packs of cigarets at a time...and outspoken. Educated at Harvard, she is highly intelligent and witty.

NOT A DANIEL

There are some who might compare Henry Kissinger with Daniel.

Daniel was among the first group of captives taken from Jerusalem to Babylon. In this matter, similar to Kissinger, he was an immigrant. Daniel within a short time, rose to become the King's right-hand man. In fact, he was so loyal to the idolatrous King, that he was trusted with the affairs of the entire empire of Babylon, and always had ready access to the palace.

Henry Kissinger, too, had a meteoric rise to world-wide fame, and became the trusted advisor of President Nixon.

However, here is where the similarity ends. Daniel was a servant of God, and bore witness to His name even in the heathen court that then ruled the entire world. In fact, he was absolutely unswerving in his own religious convictions, and did not compromise his position with idolatry.

The late J. Edgar Hoover in one of his last messages to Congress warned the lawmakers:

> The United States is Communist China's number one enemy...the most potent threat to our national security is Red China.

This statement undoubtedly made Henry Kissinger furious,

as J. Edgar Hoover made this remark prior to the President's announcement that he would visit the "People's Republic of China."

It was not unusual to discover that J. Edgar Hoover's comments were not published "for budget reasons." Soon afterward the United States recognized its No. 1 enemy!

This type of compromise with Godless nations would not have been tolerated by Daniel. Nor would Daniel have compromised his position by extensive nightlife activities.

KISSINGER, The Man

Some may conclude that Henry Kissinger delights in his playboy image, while mistrusting the feminine foundations on which it is built.

"I know their game," he once remarked. "I'm their celebrity of the hour, the new man in town."

Just what type of man is Henry Kissinger, and what are his plans for the future?

Some who have worked with him say that in his office Kissinger tends to be impatient, authoritarian, and brusque with his subordinates to the point of rudeness. This, however, may be a necessary part of **super-efficiency.**

With his superiors, he is formal and distant. He is enthusiastic in his work, and an indefatigable worker who drives himself even more brutally than he does his own subordinates.

Perhaps the key to Kissinger's diplomacy is **secrecy.** In all of his diplomatic dealings with China, Russia, and with the Arabs and Israel, one thing comes to the forefront, and that is secrecy.

A second characteristic of Henry Kissinger is his **drive.**

His whirlwind trips around the capitals of the world represent more than showmanship. They are a technique which he has developed for keeping matters constantly on the move.

Another feature of importance is that Henry Kissinger **does not seek any eternal peace** pact in his dealings. He accepts the fact of war as reality, and aims mainly to bring rival parties together. In Henry Kissinger's continued meetings with the Arabs and Israelis after the Yom Kippur War, he took a 15-day trip to thirteen countries. Every night on the trip, he sent back a ten page memo to Mr. Nixon on what he had done during the day. And without fail, he received a reply from Mr. Nixon of two to three pages in the morning giving him instructions or advice.

The Problem of Security

Security on trips for Henry Kissinger is becoming more and more difficult.

Secret Service agents often drive behind his car with submachine guns sticking out the windows. They fear an assasination attempt somewhere along the line.

When in early March, 1974 he made a visit to Syria, the State Department recorded that an assasination attempt had been inadvertently thwarted when Mr. Kissinger at the last moment cancelled a trip through the inner city of Damascus.

As he becomes more and more accessible in his dealings internationally, his security will become more and more difficult, particularly if there is some measure of success along the Arab-Israeli lines.

I'm sure there are some who are wondering that if Henry Kissinger were the victim of an assasination, whether or not he would rise again.

Henry Kissinger does not take people into his confidence very easily. In fact, he remarked to one journalist:

My success...stems from the fact that I've always acted alone.

Someone else has remarked, "Henry approaches problems like a laser beam with a fine cutting focus. This clearly gets results. But he does tend to be secretive."

About 1960, Henry Kissinger wrote a book entitled, *A World Restored: Castlereagh, Metternich, and the Problems of Peace.*

We get greater insight into Henry Kissinger when we understand that one of his heroes is Prince Von Metternich. Von Metternich was an Austrian statesman and diplomat who dominated Europe from 1814 to 1848. That period is often called, "The Age of Metternich."

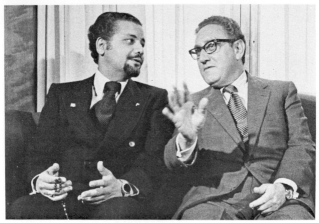

The subject was oil...or rather, the lack of oil! Secretary of State Kissinger conferring with Ahmed Zaki al-Yamani, Saudi Arabian Minister of Petroleum affairs. Sheik Yamani holds worry beads. As Americans waited in long lines in gasoline stations perhaps many of them wondered if they should be holding the worry beads!

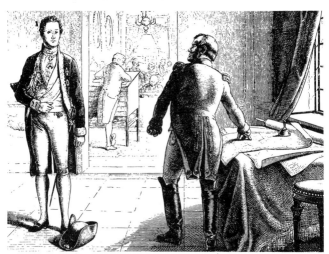

Metternich, known for his great ability at deception, convinces Napoleon, right, that Austria was neutral. But the next day Austria joined Russia against Napoleon!

It was Metternich who believed that democracy and nationalism would lead to disaster.

Prince Von Metternich met with Napoleon at Dresden on June 26, 1813, and assured him of Austrian neutrality in Europe. But the next day, Austria joined Prussia and Russia against Napoleon.

Metternich was known for his great ability at deception. And he practiced this on Napoleon. Some have said that the success of Henry Kissinger's approach to the manipulation of men and events has depended not a little upon his flair for calculated ambiguity—amounting at times to the talent for deception.

Everyone who has followed Henry Kissinger realizes that he moves about at a frenzied pace. In 1973, he travelled 120,000 miles, contacting leaders of the world. This is approximately five times around the world.

In a newspaper poll taken in Israel, he was voted the most popular person. President Nixon placed second, and Prime Minister Golda Meir ran a poor third.

A Coming World Leader?

What about Henry Kissinger the man?

From some aspects he does not have the charismatic personality one would expect of a world leader. He has a deep, monotonous voice with a very recognizable Germanic accent. In fact, in the first two years that Henry Kissinger was in the Administration, he was not placed on television, because the White House feared that his German accent would project a poor image.

At first, only silent film was permitted of him. Henry Kissinger very rarely gives interviews. By early 1974, the State Department had 275 requests for interviews with him. It is doubtful that many of them will ever be honored.

When the Gallup Poll took a survey to find out which man the American people admire most...the 1973 survey showed that Secretary of State Henry Kissinger headed the list while President Nixon fell to third place.

Perhaps one event was more responsible than any other for propelling Henry Kissinger into the forefront, even above the President of the United States. That was the Vietnam war.

Some may remember the two line poem:

**Two men looked out from prison bars,
One saw mud, the other saw stars.**

While most world leaders viewed the Vietnam War as an endless quagmire, Henry Kissinger saw not mud, but stars. Through a series of secret meetings and many conferences which had been preceeded with 42 months of talks, he was finally able to conclude what President Nixon referred to as, "peace with honor" in Southeast Asia.

On Sunday, January 28, 1973, the Vietnam cease-fire agreement was signed in Paris.

The then, Secretary of State, William P. Rogers, wrote his name 62 times on the document providing—after twelve long years—a settlement of the longest, most disheartening foreign war in American history.

This questionable peace primarily was brought about by the singular efforts of Henry Kissinger.

It is important to note the remarks of the New York Times in reporting on the peace agreement:

> *The peace agreements were as ambiguous as the conflict....The peace agreements signed today were built of compromises that permit the two Vietnamese sides to give them contradictory meanings and, they clearly hope, to continue their unfinished struggle in the political arena without continuing the slaughter.*

It was this type of peace agreement that Henry Kissinger had welded together. It was a peace agreement which was ambiguous, and one which permitted each side to give contradictory meanings to the agreement terms. This perhaps, is the key in understanding the success of Henry Kissinger's surface ability to achieve peace.

It is interesting to note that the famed Nobel Prize for that year went to Henry Kissinger and his counterpart, Le Duc Tho of North Vietnam.

Henry Kissinger willingly accepted the Nobel Prize, but Le Duc Tho did not, stating, in his own words, that peace had really not been achieved.

Peace That is no Peace

In fact, one year later, by January of 1974, it was estimated that 50,000 North and South Vietnamese had been killed in almost continuing brush fighting during the previous twelve months. In other words, as many Vietnamese had been killed since the peace one year ago, as Americans had been killed during the twelve years of war. During this same year from the signing of the peace pact it was estimated that some 800,000 new refugees had also fled from combat areas.

And the United States is still spending more than $2 Billion dollars a year to keep South Vietnam supplied with tanks, shells, planes, and bombs.

Yet President Nixon and his Number One man, Henry Kissinger, would have us believe that we have achieved "peace with honor" in Vietnam.

Arsenal Of Power

Part of Henry Kissinger's ability to negotiate is the realization that the United States possesses formidable weaponry that has the power to destroy the entire world. The Defense Department budget within a year or two should rise to about $85 Billion annually. Or an increase of $6 Billion over the 1974 estimate.

Henry Kissinger knows that expenditures by military and aerospace agencies on laser arms are expected to average over $300 million annually for the next five years. These new weapons are revolutionary in nature, in their ability to destroy effectively weapons of the enemy.

Among the $3.3 Billion of new weapons in the arsenal of Death are included: a new battletank, to replace the M-60 tank; a complex surface-to-air missile, designed to hit enemy planes swooping in low over ground troops; and star scopes, which magnify the light available on even the darkest night more than 50,000 times, and provide night scouts with a noon-time view of a target. This object is mounted atop rifles and other weaponry.

Also included are mines, which are smaller than a soldier's hand, that can be strewn in front of an advancing enemy like confetti; and bigger and vastly more powerful and controversial nuclear mines.

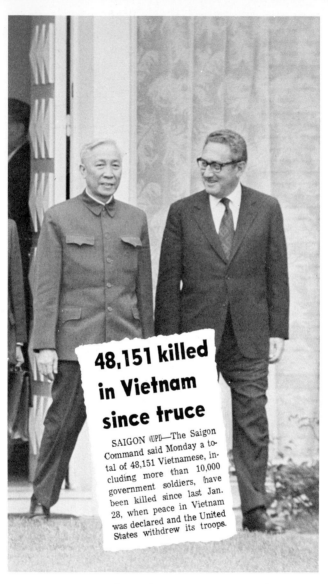

48,151 killed in Vietnam since truce

SAIGON (UPI)—The Saigon Command said Monday a total of 48,151 Vietnamese, including more than 10,000 government soldiers, have been killed since last Jan. 28, when peace in Vietnam was declared and the United States withdrew its troops.

Henry Kissinger with North Vietnam's Le Duc Tho emerging from one of many peace meetings near Paris.

Henry Kissinger also realizes that the Pentagon is doing far-out research in the development of computers that speak and understand conversational English, computers that can "see" just as humans do, and computers that can make political decisions as well as anticipate the actions of foreign governments. This is all being done under the Defense Advanced Research Projects Agency, (ARPA), which has an overall budget of over $200 million a year.

The potential ability of these advanced computers is frightening. **And all of this knowledge is in the hands of Henry Kissinger.**

PEACE MAKER of the MIDDLE EAST

October 6, 1973 will be a date that will be long remembered, for this was to be Henry Kissinger's biggest crisis, and greatest challenge.

It was on that date that Egyptian forces crossed the Suez Canal into Israeli-occupied Sinai Peninsula, and thus began an eruption of the heaviest fighting in the Middle East since the 1967 war.

At the same time, the Syrian troops launched a drive south of the Golan Heights. This attack came on Yom Kippur as Jews were celebrating the holiest day in their calendar.

Perhaps the oddest thing about the entire war and the subsequent cooling off period between the Jews and the Arabs is that the chief negotiator for the settlement was himself a Jew—Henry Kissinger.

In an off-the-cuff remark, Henry Kissinger himself said that one of the odder barometers of our relations with Israel and the Arab world is, "Who's kissing Kissinger?"

When Kissinger attended a reception hosted by Israeli defense minister Moshe Dayan, he told a Tel Aviv newspaper reporter that Arabs were friendlier than Jews.

> *Every time my plane lands in an Arab capital, I am welcomed with a kiss on both cheeks. But, (foreign minister) Abba Eban has never given me the least little kiss.*

Israel suffered greatly during the Yom Kippur War. For them this war was not the same success as the Six-Day war, and the mood of the people had changed—wearied by 25 years of conflict.

Sometimes we become so engulfed with the details of the Yom Kippur War and its ensuing results that we fail to realize the magnificent coup that Henry Kissinger was able to achieve through his diplomatic negotiations done in secret. Only time can tell whether deception entered into such negotiations.

But a quotation from THE TIMES OF ISRAEL, April 1974 issue, gives some reflection as to one of Henry Kissinger's most astounding successes and Israel's dependence on this one man:

> *In a sense, everybody's gambling on Henry Kissinger. The guts of the disengagement pact— the so-called U.S. Proposal limiting Egypt to 7,000 men and 30 tanks on the east bank of the canal and no SAM missiles within 8 miles of the west bank—is an Egyptian-U.S. agreement, after all, not an Egyptian-Israeli agreement...The fact is, the U.S. has gone to special pains to emphasize that it does not 'guarantee' the accord, that the entire agreement is based on 'trust'....*

Whatever else it is, it must have been terribly persuasive! Kissinger got Israel to pull back to the Mitla Pass without so much as a declaration of peaceful intent on Sadat's part!

For this, Israel surrendered her own bridgehead on the west bank, broke the encirclement of the third Egyptian corps, and handed Egypt undisputed control of the east bank!

Even Yigal Allon (Deputy Premier of Israel) had to concede that in bald geographical terms it was a "unilateral Israeli withdrawal."

Imagine if you can, the fact that the Israeli Army was already on Egyptian territory, and within a matter of days could have entered Cairo, and conquered Egypt. Yet, in effect, this one man, Henry Kissinger was able to convince Israel to stop her advance and without any real concessions on the part of Egypt, to pull back from the encirclement.

Only a Henry Kissinger could have accomplished such a coup!

At no time in recent history has anyone been able to achieve so quickly a semblance of peace in the Middle East, but Henry Kissinger did it within an extremely short span of time.

Those of us who are familiar with Bible prophecy know that according to Daniel 9:27 there will be a time in the future when another man of peace will be able to achieve what will seem to be the impossible, and that is, the final bringing of the Arabs and Jews together under a semblance of peace.

Could this successful action on the part of Henry Kissinger be a prototype of what others will witness at the start of the Tribulation Period when Antichrist is able to achieve a similar, but more effective agreement? Only time will tell, but we are witnessing a pattern being established that is drawing us closer to the End Times.

KISSINGER...Whirlwind of PEACE

Actually Henry Kissinger has been able to meet almost anyone that he has set his mind to meet.

Only one important individual refused to meet with him. That was the Palestinian terrorist leader Yasser Arafat, who turned down a request to meet with Secretary of State Henry Kissinger in December 1973. Arafat's associate told a group of students that Kissinger was a "Zionist...a more Zionist man cannot be found."

When Defense Minister Moshe Dayan spoke with Henry Kissinger for two hours, Henry Kissinger had so convinced him that a compromise was needed, that Dayan stated, "We feel we want to make peace, to make compromises...."

It was Secretary of State Henry Kissinger's insistent prodding that finally brought a disengagement of Arab-Israeli forces engaged in the Yom Kippur War, and the Mid East compromise that followed in January 1974.

"Insistent prodding" would be a mild name perhaps, for what occurred, because Mr. Kissinger was certainly insistent on achieving a conclusion to his negotiations.

In fact, he travelled so frequently between Egypt and Israel, that one night Under Secretary of State, Joseph J. Sisco, stood in the aisle of the Air Force jet prior to its

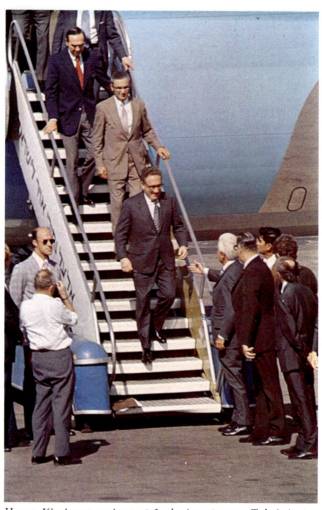

Henry Kissinger arrives at Lod airport near Tel Aviv to begin a long series of negotiations relative to the Yom Kippur War.

taking off, and shouted, "Welcome aboard the Egyptian-Israeli shuttle!"

This was after hopping for four consecutive days between Aswan and Tel Aviv.

KISSINGER...The Tattered Peace

Both Premier Golda Meir and Moshe Dayan have been impressed by Henry Kissinger's abilities to negotiate. In fact, Mr. Dayan stated that no previous intermediary was as good in trying to reach an Arab-Israeli settlement as Henry Kissinger.

But many Israelis find it hard to accept the situation when an American Secretary of State, who is a Jew, is welcomed by such long time enemies of Israel as King Faisal of Saudi Arabia.

One senior Israeli official commented, "Kissinger has a dazzling smile...but there are gaps in it—and there are gaps in this agreement, big enough for the whole thing to fall through."

But when Kissinger returned to the United States he was hailed as an apostle of peace. Cartoonists for the Miami Daily News pictured Henry Kissinger as a Moses with his ten commandments coming down from the mountain.

Perhaps Kissinger's next move will be to urge Israel to withdraw to its pre-June 1967 War borders. If he were able to achieve this, Henry Kissinger believes that Saudi Arabia would boost its oil production to 20 million barrels a day —once the United States could guarantee an Israeli pull-back behind the 1967 boundaries. This would be more than twice the 8 million barrels that came out of Saudi oil fields each day before the Yom Kippur War. If he were able to achieve this brilliant maneuver, he would not only have the Arabs on his side, but the majority of the American public who are tired of waiting in long lines to get gasoline!

Many Israelis feel that Henry Kissinger has forgotten his origins, and forgotten the persecution of his countrymen by Hitler.

Golda Meir bitterly remembers Neville Chamberlain's trip to the Munich Conference, and the ensuing disastrous World War II, and she hasn't hesitated in reminding

Kissinger of this event, and that history has a habit of repeating itself.

In perhaps the most prophetically-aligned commentary of the entire war, was a picture of Henry Kissinger on the front cover of THE JERUSALEM POST magazine, January 18, 1974, which was titled, "Henry, the Peacemaker."

Only time will tell how prophetically significant another ad was. On November 30, 1973, in THE JERUSALEM POST, an ad appeared by the Citizens for Prevention of a National Disaster, which in part read:

> Don't remain silent! Fight Kissinger's pressures!

It continued in part:

> We know that ruthless Kissinger pressure denied us the completion of the military victory due any people subjected to a vicious sneak attack....As Jews and loyal Americans, your duty is to arouse America for the desperate fight against the Kissinger (Chamberlain) policy of appeasing aggressors.

> We are greatly ashamed and concerned over Kissinger's exploitation of his own supposed Jewish loyalties, as the means to lure us into his trap of appeasement.

A reproduction of this entire ad appears in this book.

KISSINGER'S COMPROMISE — RUSSIA'S GAIN

One thing that Henry Kissinger achieved for the Egyptians goes almost unnoticed by many, and yet it is this singular achievement which may be the tool that will spell tragedy for Israel in the future.

Israel, under the terms of the peace, agreed to pull back east of the Suez Canal. By so doing, for the first time in nearly seven years, the world's greatest man-made water-way was once again under Egyptian control. And immediately President Anwar Sadat charted a visionary program for an ambitious canal project that dwarfs the original scheme of its builder, Ferdinand De Lesseps.

Egyptian plans are to expand the Suez Canal to four times its original size, enabling today's super tankers once more to sail through the desert. At the same time, they plan to make one million acres of the desert "blossom as a rose" through a massive irrigation scheme.

But aside from that, and more important—the canal will enable the Soviet Navy to move warships more easily into the Indian Ocean, and perhaps give the Kremlin a strategic advantage over the United States in controlling the entire Middle East.

The Greatest Challenge

Then in late February 1974, Secretary of State Kissinger pulled another rabbit out of the hat. All he did was get Syria and Egypt to agree to talk disengagement...but this very act broke up a 25 year Mid East stalemate! Under Henry Kissinger's persistent pressure, now at last, most Arab governments are resigned to talking to Israel.

Even Libya's President Qaddafi joined the parade. After Henry Kissinger gets them to talk, his next step will be to get everyone to Geneva. His most troublesome problem to settle will be the Palestinian Arab Refugee question. As the obstacles get tougher, it will be interesting to see how Henry Kissinger is able to resolve each stalemate.

The Palestinian question will not be an easy one to resolve. It is estimated that three million Palestinians live in Arab lands or in Israel and Israeli-occupied territories.

The refugee camps where 644,000 Palestinians live breed violence and hatred. These are people without a country to turn to—a people who have lived 25 years without hope.

Now the Geneva Conference holds out a shred of hope. What are the issues? They are simple. The Palestinians say there must be a secular state of Arabs and Jews in what used to be Palestine—no Zionist Israel continually invading the land with more Jews from all over the world.

The Israelis say that they are willing to turn some territory back to the Palestinians—but they will accept no independent state of Palestine on their borders or within them.

Now it's up to Henry Kissinger! And this will be a tough nut to crack, because there is no agreement among the Arabs themselves about the rights of the Palestinians, and there is certainly no agreement among the Palestinians.

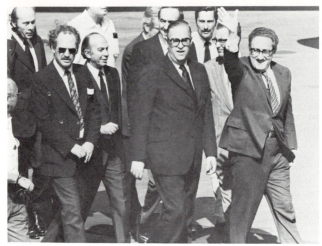

Henry Kissinger arrives at Tel Aviv during sensitive negotiations to end Yom Kippur War. Left of Kissinger is Israel's Foreign Minister Abba Eban.

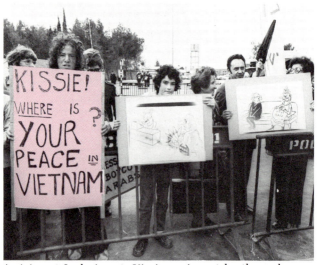

Arriving at Lod airport, Kissinger is met by these demonstrators protesting what they believe to be a pro-Arab settlement.

And what about the fate of Jerusalem? Henry Kissinger has seen almost every major leader of the world. As of this writing, however, he has not yet met the Pope. And it is Pope Paul who has urged that Jerusalem should not be under the exclusive control of any one religion, but should be under a guardianship, where the Pope himself would have a voice on the future of Jerusalem and the holy places.

It will be interesting to see what, if anything, Secretary of State Henry Kissinger does to resolve the problem of Jerusalem.

AN UNEASY EUROPE

Henry Kissinger's restless diplomacy irritates the Europeans.

They don't know quite what to make of him, and his success in Europe has not been as great as has his success in China, and in the Middle East.

Henry Kissinger is not interested in talking to individual European leaders as much as he is interested in talking to a United Europe. **It would appear that his greatest desire is to see Europe united as a single unit of government.**

In December 1973, Henry Kissinger made a special trip to Europe covering five countries, meeting with NATO and Common Market leaders.

After the meeting, a European diplomat commented:

> Kissinger will always play with us. It's his temperment. He tries to convince us that we have to shut up and let him handle things on our behalf....

Henry Kissinger is always looking for new horizons and when he addressed the Common Market Nations in December 1973, he remarked:

> With whomever I will speak among my colleagues, I will stress that the Atlantic Alliance remains the cornerstone of American foreign policy, but I shall also emphasize a new act of vision is necessary so that it can remain the cornerstone of our common endeavors.

As one Israeli official commented:

> Kissinger operates with promises, he explains the other side's position and what your choices are....

Oftentimes the choices leave nothing to choose, and Henry Kissinger again achieves a successful settlement from what might have been a bitter confrontation.

After resolving the Middle East crisis, and soothing the feathers of Europe's Common Market, he flew to Mexico City in February 1974 in his first major venture into Latin American policy. He came to seek a solution to the delicate problem of United States investments abroad.

The theme of his message to the 24 Latin American and Caribbean nations was, "We need each other."

However, Mr. Kissinger's ideas were greeted with skepticism as many remarked, "...promises—and more promises!"

It will be a test of Mr. Kissinger's skill if he is able to convince Latin America that the United States is honestly interested in their welfare.

One Israeli writer commented in a recent issue of THE JERUSALEM POST that:

> Dr. Kissinger's moves in the Middle East are a dangerous folly...Every American 'achievement' in Cairo is a step towards strengthening the Arab-Soviet cooperation.

> To convince Jerusalem, Kissinger used an interchanging system of threats and promises. Some of the threats turned out to be hollow and several of his promises were not fulfilled, but the system in general is still effective.

And quite prophetically, the writer of this article stated, "For Israel, giving in will only be a gradual Holocaust."

A UNITED STATES of EUROPE?

One of Henry Kissinger's greatest desires is to resolve the problems of world energy. Thus at the 13 nation energy conference held in Washington in February 1974, Henry Kissinger offered a seven-point program of cooperation. This was to be a "truly massive joint effort," by oil consumers and producers to overcome the world energy crisis and preserve the international economic order.

His message that day clearly appealed for unity among

the cooperative nations, when he ended his talk by saying,

> We confront a fundamental decision. Will we
> consume ourselves in nationalistic rivalry which
> the realities of interdependence makes suicidal?
> Or will we acknowledge our interdependence and
> shape cooperative solutions?

Cooperative solutions? What does this mean and what will it entail? Does Henry Kissinger see at some far distant point as his solution, the unification of European states into a Common Market? Or does he foresee a United States of Europe in which the United States and Europe will blend its powers? And does he see himself as having some highly powerful position as the moving force at the head of such a unification?

We do not know, and perhaps even at this time, he does not know.

But the surface successes that he has had could certainly be the preparatory ground that would pave the way for such a position. If, as somewhat alleged, Prince Metternich is the idol of Henry Kissinger...then it would be well to look into some of the statements made by Prince Metternich in the 1800's.

Among them were the following:

> In Europe, democracy is a falsehood.

He had doubts of its permanence even in America, and said:

> I do not know where it will end, but it cannot end
> in a quiet old age.

Napoleon said of Metternich:

> He is almost a statesman: he lies well.

Talleyrand made the following comparison between Mazarin, a French statesman and Cardinal, and Metternich:

> The Cardinal deceived, but did not lie: now Prince
> Metternich always lies, but never deceives.

To what can we attribute Henry Kissinger's apparent successes, achieved with meteoric speed? Can it be attributed to his background of scholarly education? Can it be attributed to a carefully conceived, intricate plan of strategy that he prepares before he enters each arena of negotiation? Are his successes achieved through human abilities? Or, is there some mysterious force that propels this one man so singularly to achieve so much in so short a time?

Only time can reveal this.

The Number 666

Ever since Henry Kissinger's rise to prominence in world affairs, I have been flooded with phone calls and letters concerning this man.

Some people have called me claiming to have special visions. Others have met me personally, and in confidential terms expressed that they had the key to the answer of who Antichrist was.

In each case, the individual was certain that Antichrist was Henry Kissinger. Some have constructed elaborate number-letter charts based on the Bible verse, Revelation 13:18 which reads:

Here is wisdom. Let him that hath understanding count the number of the beast [Antichrist]; for it is the number of a man; and his number is Six hundred three score and six.

Some have come up with the following numerical chart to buttress their conclusion that Henry Kissinger is the Antichrist.

It, however, would be both unfair and unwise for any Christian at this time to label Henry Kissinger as Antichrist —for who knows, perhaps your name too adds up to 666?

The chart starts at A and increases each letter by 6

		The Name & Number
A - 6	N - 84	
B - 12	O - 90	
C - 18	P - 96	**K** - 66
D - 24	Q - 102	**I** - 54
E - 30	R - 108	**S** - 114
F - 36	S - 114	**S** - 114
G - 42	T - 120	**I** - 54
H - 48	U - 126	**N** - 84
I - 54	V - 132	**G** - 42
J - 60	W - 138	**E** - 30
K - 66	X - 144	**R** - 108
L - 72	Y - 150	666
M - 78	Z - 156	

However it must be kept in mind that this same type of numbering system has been used in the past to show that others, including the Pope of Rome, is to be the Antichrist.

One title of the Pope of Rome is Vicarivs Filii Dei. If you take the letters of his title which represent Latin numerals (printed large) and add them together, they come to **666** as per the computation listed below.

V -	5	F -	0
I -	1	I -	1
C -	100	L -	50
A -	0	I -	1
R -	0	I -	1
I -	1		
V -	5	D -	500
S -	0	E -	0
		I -	1
			666

Christmastide, 1973

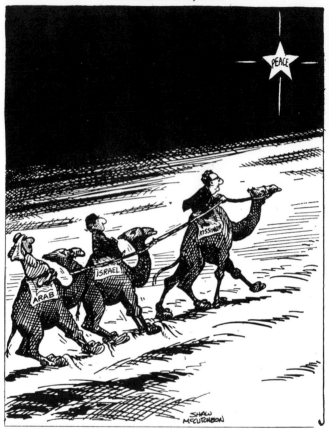

Others have said that **666** applies to Pope Paul VI:

PAUL VI = 6 letters in his name
Paul in latin is Paulus. This is also 6 letters.
He was the 6th Pope named Paul

Thus, **666**

His ELECTION was on 6/21/63
(This involves 2 6's and 2+1+3 = 6)

Thus, **666**

At age 66, he was the 6th Pope elected in the 20th century.

Therefore, **666**

His crowning took place on 6/30/63
(Again, 2 6's and 3 + 3 = 6)

Therefore, **666**

While Pope Paul VI was in office, the traditional mass of the Catholic Church was changed to a "new order of Mass." This change brought a split in the church.

The important thing to remember is that at this present time, **nobody knows who Antichrist is,** and certainly no Christian will know.

The Antichrist will not be known for certain as the Antichrist until the middle of the Tribulation Period (after the Rapture) when his human identity will at last be revealed. Matthew 24:15 shows this to be so.

RAPTURE COUNTDOWN Beginning

One can observe that there is a pattern being established which does indicate that we are living in the Last Days. Certainly Henry Kissinger's ability to achieve a semblance of peace and détente (a relaxation of international tension between governments) does represent a very significant milestone in history.

We do see a pattern being developed towards the fulfillment of prophecy in the End Times.

This pattern began with Israel becoming a nation in 1948; with Jerusalem at last becoming a part of Israel in 1967; with enmity against Israel by nations throughout the world in 1973; and in 1974 a whirlwind courier of peace being

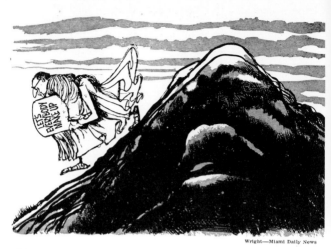

Wright—Miami Daily News

able to temporarily resolve conflicts with the major nations of the world.

Looking back over the years it would be hard to find anyone who has duplicated the spectacular achievements that have been associated with Henry Kissinger.

His persistence in negotiation enabled the United States to extricate itself out of a long, disastrous war in Vietnam. Anyone who has had any experience with the Asian culture will realize that the most complex type of negotiation is to try to achieve an agreement with an Asian nation.

He topped this success with getting the United States government to recognize one of our bitterest foes, Red China, and then capped it with having the President of the United States make a personal, official visit to Red China, and to meet not only with Chou En-Lai but also with Chairman Mao.

Henry Kissinger's diplomatic abilities come to the forefront during times of conflict because they give him the opportunity to exercise his ability to bring out of conflict, an aura of peace.

No sooner had he concluded these Asian achievements, when he was flying to the Middle East and shuttling back and forth as much as two or three times a day between Arab nations and the country of Israel in order to bring the Yom Kippur War to a conclusion.

The AMERICAN MAGICIAN

No wonder the Egyptians now refer to Henry Kissinger as, "The American Magician."

His shuttle diplomacy seems to be working. In fact, in March 1974, as the Jordanian Arab Army band marched past Secretary of State Henry A. Kissinger, before his departure from Amman, a member of the Kissinger party shook his head and said:

> It's crazy, isn't it? An Arab king honoring a Jewish-American official, with his British-style band, playing its Scottish bagpipes to a desert background.

The newsman next to him added:

> And to complete the day, in a few hours, Kissinger will be greeted by the country which he fled from 36 years ago.

What does the future hold?

God has already mapped out in the Bible the major items in His plan for the future. While we know His plan, we do not know exactly which men on earth will be the leaders involved in the terrors of the Tribulation Period.

From all indications, the rapidity of events in the last two years should be sufficient warning to Christians to double their efforts to evangelize the lost—it should also be sufficient warning to those who do not know Christ as their personal Savior to seek eternal life.

While the Egyptians may refer to Henry Kissinger as, "The American Magician," it should be evident that the problems of this present world cannot be resolved, and will not be resolved through man's efforts.

The energy crisis is a case in point.

There will come a day, however, when a so-called "Magician" will rise and fool the world into believing he has resolved the problems of our planet.

And temporarily, he will have.

Henry Kissinger—the American Magician? Only time will tell!

Arabs Fear Invasion by U.S.

Nixon W...

Pope bids for voice in fate of Jerusalem

By PEGGY POLK

VATICAN CITY (UPI). — Pope Paul VI wrote in a private memo before making his 1964 pilgrimage to the Holy Land that he hoped the visit would reawaken Roman Catholic desire for "guardianship" over its most sacred shrines, the official Vatican newspaper said

to ensure... any possible...
and th...
cies of...
from a...
The...
Africa...
peror...

Mideast Awaits Kissinger Again

Inquirer Wire Services

... Secretary of State ... Kissinger may visit ... e East within the ... ays to prod Israel ... into completing a ... r separating ...

These sources also s... they expect Kissinger, t... chief architect of the Gene... conference, to ...

Amendment Would Let Kissinger Be President

Washington— (AP) —A constitutional amendment has been proposed by Rep. Jonathan Bingham (D-NY) to allow foreign-born, naturalized U.S. citizens to be President.

Only natural-born U.S. citizens may be President under the Constitution. Bingham says that should be changed to allow someone like Secretary of State Henry A. Kissinger run for the White House. Kissinger immigrated to the United States from Germany as a child.

DAY, APRIL 11, 1974 —

GOLDA MEIR QUITS AND BRINGS DOWN CABINET IN ISRAEL

New Election Likely in 3 to 5 Months—Government Will Stay as Caretaker

DECISION CALLED FINAL

Kissinger to Visit Syria, 5 Other Mideast Nations

By MARILYN BERGER
Washington Post Service

WASHINGTON. — The State Department announced Tuesday the itinerary for Henry A. Kissinger's trip to the Mideast. It will include a stop in Damascus, the first visit to

ment officials said, would be to prepare for the peace conference that will bring Arabs and Israelis to face-to-face talks.

A major effort is expected to get Syria to release the approximately 13 Israeli prisoners of war. Israeli Foreign

Jordan, Dec. 15 and 16; Beirut, Dec. 16; Tel Aviv, Dec. 15 and 17.

Although not part of the official announcement, the swing through the Mideast—Kissinger's second in five weeks—will follow several

Antichrist

THE MAN OF PEACE
WHOSE AIMS ARE DESTRUCTION

His Character, A Friend to the Jew and Gentile • His First Move • The Reign of Antichrist • The Sequence of Events • Who is Antichrist

One of these days some great leader, admired by the world as a man of peace will offer to settle the Arab-Israeli dispute.

Watch out when this event happens. For this man will be what the Scriptures term **Antichrist.**

And his sweet words of peace will soon lead to the most devastating seven years of terror, trials, and wholesale murders. This 7-year time period will occur <u>after</u> the **Rapture**[1]. It will be known as the **Tribulation Period**[2].

The **Antichrist** is a part of the Satanic Trinity just as **Christ** is part of the Heavenly Trinity.

It is important that we know the definition before we get further into the subject.

Just as the Heavenly Trinity is made up of the:
1. Father
2. Son
3. Holy Spirit,

---

[1]
RAPTURE
This refers to the time, <u>prior</u> to the start of the 7-year Tribulation Period, when believing Christians (both dead and alive) will *"in the twinkling of an eye"* rise up to meet Christ in the air. Read 1 Thessalonians 4:13-17 in the New Testament.

[2]
TRIBULATION PERIOD
This will be a period of 7 years, <u>following</u> the Rapture, of phenomenal world trial and suffering. It is at this time that Antichrist will reign over a federation of 10 nations which quite possibly could include the Common Market nations and the United States. See Daniel 9:27 and Matthew 24:21.

so likewise in the counterfeit Trinity the members are:

1. Satan
   He is sometimes referred in the Scriptures as the Dragon and is known as anti-God. He imitates the work of God the Father (Revelation 12:9; 20:2).

2. Antichrist
   He is sometimes referred in the Scriptures as the Beast. Antichrist imitates the work of God the Son (Revelation 13:1; 19:20).

3. The False Prophet
   He is sometimes referred in the Scriptures as the Second Beast. The False Prophet imitates the work of God the Holy Spirit (Revelation 13:11; 19:20).

The word **Antichrist** means an enemy of Christ or one who usurps Christ's name and authority.

As you may recall, 2 Thessalonians 2:1-12 refers to the Antichrist as "that man of sin" and states that he will oppose and exalt himself above God and will actually sit in the temple of God and claim to be God.

ANTICHRIST AND THE FALSE PROPHET

Both the Antichrist and the False Prophet will be living during what is termed as the Tribulation Period.

This Tribulation Period will last for seven years. The second 3½ years especially will be filled with terror, death and destruction.

The False Prophet, however, does not try to promote himself and should not be confused with the Antichrist.

The False Prophet never becomes an object of worship. He does the work of a prophet by directing attention away from himself and towards the Antichrist whom he says has the right to be worshipped (Revelation 13:12).

Both the Antichrist and the False Prophet are tools in the hands of Satan and their every move will be guided by Satan.

It is quite interesting to note that Jesus Christ in John 5:43 seems to have made a prophetic reference to the Antichrist when He said:

> "I am come in my Father's name, and ye receive me not: if another shall come in his own name, him ye will receive."

It is also sad to reflect that the Jews rejected Jesus Christ as their Messiah—but when the Antichrist comes they will be deceived by him and accept him and welcome him with open arms as their king and saviour.

In Daniel 11:36, 37 we are told that the Antichrist will "...exalt himself, and magnify himself above every god...."

And in 2 Thessalonians 2:4 it is revealed, "...so that he as God sitteth in the temple of God, shewing himself that he is God."

There are indications in the Bible that Antichrist will become popular because of the prevailing lawlessness that occurs throughout the world and his **supposed ability** to resolve world problems.

HIS CHARACTER (Revelation 13)
A FRIEND TO THE JEW AND GENTILE

Antichrist will be an extremely popular individual. He will pose as a great humanitarian and the friend of men. **He will appear to be a very special friend to the Jewish race.** There is no doubt from the Scriptures that he will persuade the Jews that he has come to usher in the golden age for the Jewish race. In light of this they will receive him as their Messiah.

> One might say that he is a "composite man" who will have an irresistible personality. Because of his versatile accomplishments, super-human wisdom, and great administrative and executive ability he will be looked upon with favor by all of the world leaders and populace.

Along with his powers as a brilliant diplomat he will be a superb strategist in the art of war.

Keep in mind that this Antichrist will come into prominence during the Tribulation Period. At the moment of the Rapture, there will not be left one single believer on this earth.

So basically at the beginning of the Tribulation Period, everyone on the earth will be an unbeliever and look to this Antichrist with great fascination and believe that he offers the world life-saving salvation.

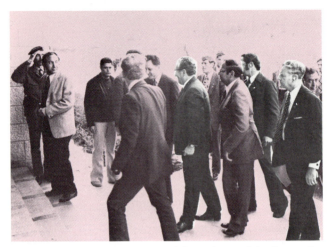

Henry Kissinger, accompanied by a host of bodyguards, enters Golda Meir's office for negotiations. Note radio earphones in two guards at right.

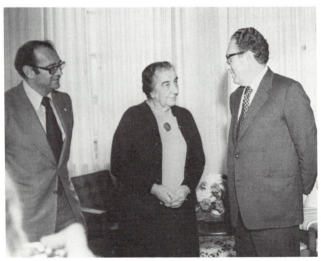

Henry Kissinger meets with Premier Golda Meir during Yom Kippur War crisis.

One thing is certain from the many references found regarding the Antichrist in the Scriptures: He will be a counterfeit and a clever imitation of a true Christ.

> His rise will be sudden.
> This also will be an imitation of Christ.

You will recall that Christ for 30 years remained in obscurity in his home in Nazareth and the silence of those years is broken only once in Luke 2.

Comparatively, the Antichrist will also remain in obscurity and then suddenly his rise will be brought into prominence. He may even now be in the world and preparing for his Satan-directed work.

HE PROMISES PEACE

As was stated before, undoubtedly one of the elements of his marvelous success in gaining the hearts of the people lies in the fact that he will come promising the very thing that is uppermost in the hearts of people all over the world today: PEACE!

This man, in the person of Antichrist, will accomplish this very thing . . . but what most people do not realize is that this accomplishment will be only for a little season—and then the very gates of Hell will break loose here on earth.

HIS FIRST MOVE

One of the first moves of the Antichrist will be to gain the confidence of the Jewish people and others by his diplomatically settling the then explosive Middle East situation.

Therefore, his first attempt is to gain the favor of the Jewish people.

After accomplishing this, he will help the Jewish people immeasurably probably by returning many of them to the land of Israel and he will show them many favors.

Actually the Tribulation Period will begin with a public appearance of Antichrist when he participates in the making of a significant seven year Middle East peace pact (Daniel 9:27). At this time, however, he will not yet be recognized as the Antichrist. This recognition awaits another 3½ years (Matthew 24:15).

Henry Kissinger
Man on the move !

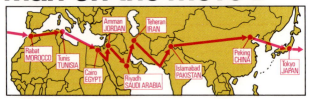

The November 1973 Whirlwind Tour of Henry Kissinger

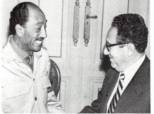

Kissinger with Egypt's Anwar Sadat

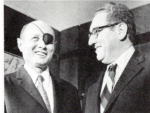

with Israel's Moshe Dayan

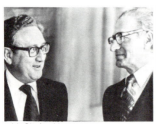

with Shah of Iran

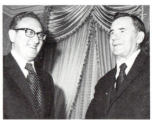

with Russia's Andrei Gromyko

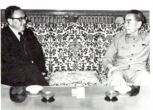

with China's Chou En-Lai

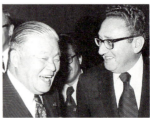

with Japan's Masayoshi Ohira

This individual will eventually be the head of what may be known as the Federated States of Europe. As the head of this organization, he would be able to exert great authority and power by attempting to settle the Arab-Israeli dispute.

The Scriptures seem to indicate that he will side with Israel in backing her claim to the land of Palestine.

Russia will be a part of a northern confederacy and will back the Arab's claim to Palestine.

The following verses in 2 Thessalonians 2 and Ezekiel 38 exhibit this prophecy.

> And thou (Russia) shalt come from thy place out of the north parts . . . all of them riding upon horses . . . a mighty army: And thou shalt come up against my people of Israel . . . surely in that day there shall be a great shaking in the land of Israel (Ezekiel 38:15,16,19).

> And then shall that Wicked (Antichrist) be revealed, whom the Lord shall consume with the spirit of his mouth . . . whose coming is after the working of Satan with all power and signs and lying wonders (2 Thessalonians 2:8,9).

It is estimated today that there are some 3 million Jews living in Israel.

To some extent they are reviving many of their distinctive historic features and customs. However, surveys show that the religious faith of the vast majority of Jews is neither Biblical Judaism nor Christianity.

Most of them hold to a liberalized Judaism religion and some of them, as in the case of so many of today's population, are even atheists.

There are very few Jews in Israel who accept Jesus Christ as the true Messiah or look to God literally to fulfill Old Testament prophecies.

In spite of this, however, they still look upon the land of Palestine as the country of great promise for them.

Why would Russia want to invade Palestine or Israel?

Scientists have discovered that all of the manufactured goods, fruits and vegetables exported from this land of

Israel are nothing in comparison with the mineral wealth of the Dead Sea.

Since the days of Abraham which were four thousands of years ago, God has been pouring into this mysterious sea a fabulous amount of wealth in the form of mineral salts.

Only with the return of the Jews to this land, have attempts been made to discover the mineral content of the Dead Sea. The analysis shows that the value of the chemicals in the Dead Sea is $1,270,000,000,000. It is believed that this staggering sum is equal to the combined wealth of the United States, Great Britain, France, Germany and Italy.

THE REIGN OF ANTICHRIST

As we stated before, the Antichrist will continue to rise for 3½ years and then he will reign for 3½ years (Revelation 13:5). This is the length of the Tribulation Period. He will be President of the 10 Federated Nations. These nations may be known as the Federated States of Europe.

While it is true that at present the great problem facing the Western powers today is the problem of trying to bring together, under the same head, nations that were originally part of the same Roman Empire . . . this problem will be erased in the near future.

The 10 Federated States of Europe will probably include France, England and Germany (Possibly West Germany) as well as lesser countries, and perhaps the United States.

The prophecy is revealed in Revelation (17:12-13), which shows that these nations that were once a part of the Roman Empire will gather together and are going to enter into an agreement to give their authority to one man as their head (Daniel 7:7-8,23-26 compared with Rev. 13).

This one man will be the Antichrist.

THE MAN OF PEACE BECOMES THE MAN OF WAR

To those in Israel, the first 3½ years will seem like a heaven on earth.

They are back in their land. The Antichrist has fulfilled his promises in bringing peace to the land and protecting the Jews from the onrushing armies of Russia and her allies.

Jerusalem is looked up to as one of the most elite cities of the world and is the hub of business activity, fashion and world culture.

It would appear that Utopia had arrived. At last the world could now settle down to a world of peace under the protectorate of a great world leader who has amassed under him the cooperation of the 10 powerful states known as the European Federation of States.

But the honeymoon soon will be over and the next 3½ years (the last half of the Tribulation Period) ushers in a most horrible period of death and destruction for both the Jews and those who then will turn to Christ.

How does this all begin and why does it occur?

THE SEQUENCE OF EVENTS

Now let's look at the sequence of the events. When does all of this take place?

The Antichrist will make this convenant with the nation Israel at the very beginning of the Tribulation Period. He will come claiming to be the great man of peace and he will guarantee peace for Israel. He appears to make a seven year peace compact involving Israel which he then proceeds to honor for the first 3½ years of the Tribulation (Daniel 9:27).

After the Antichrist as head of the Federated States of Europe secures the land of Palestine for Israel, Russia seems to start her forces working to overtake this land. But Russia will be defeated.[3] Behind the scenes maneuvering will probably take between 2 and 3 years during the first 3½ year segment of this Tribulation Period.

WHY GOD ALLOWS
THE TRIBULATION PERIOD TO OCCUR

Israel had been warned that this Tribulation event would occur. In the Old Testament, these prophecies were predicted in Isaiah, Daniel, and Jeremiah.

[3]

For a comprehensive description of the events that lead up to the Tribulation Period and the Tribulation Period, we suggest you read **GUIDE TO SURVIVAL** by Salem Kirban. $1.95.

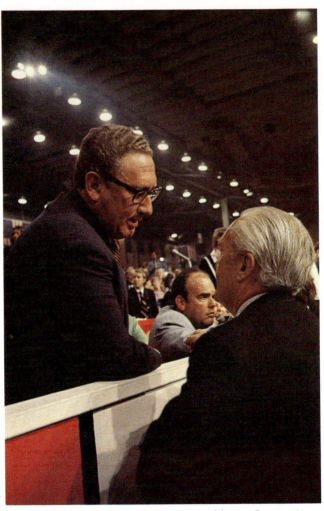

Henry Kissinger at 1972 Miami Republican Convention. Man seated is former Assistant to the President, John D. Ehrlichman.

Even the Lord Jesus, Himself, had told what was coming and what the Jews would do at that time.

> I am come in my Father's name, and ye receive me not: if another shall come in his own name, him ye will receive (John 5:43).

Let's look at the comparison. Jesus had come without deception, claiming to be sent by His Father.

> For I came down from heaven, not to do mine own will, but the will of him that sent me. (38)

> And this is the Father's will which hath sent me, that of all which He hath given me I should lose nothing, but should raise it up again at the last day (39) (John 6:38-39).

He gave all the glory to His Father.

> And, behold, one came and said unto him, Good Master, what good thing shall I do, that I may have eternal life? (16)

> And he said unto him, Why callest thou me good? there is none good but one, that is, God: but if thou wilt enter into life, keep the commandments (17) (Matthew 19:16-17).

> But if I do, though ye believe not me, believe the works: that ye may know, and believe, that the Father is in me, and I in him (John 10:38).

And yet, Jesus warned the Jews that there would be one coming who would claim to be God and demand worship as such.

It is during this second 3 1/2 year period of the Tribulation, this man of sin, Antichrist, will be revealed.

He is the incarnation of Satan himself.

> And his power shall be mighty, but not by his own power: and he shall destroy wonderfully, and shall prosper, and practise, and shall destroy the mighty and the holy people (Daniel 8:24).

This will be Satan's supreme effort.

> Therefore rejoice, ye heavens, and ye that dwell in them. Woe to the inhabiters of the earth and of

> the sea! for the devil is come down unto you,
> having great wrath, because he knoweth that he
> hath but a short time (Revelation 12:12).

And for this he had schemed thousands of years.

> How art thou fallen from heaven, O Lucifer
> (Satan), son of the morning! how art thou cut
> down to the ground, which didst weaken the
> nations! (12)

> For thou hast said in thine heart, I will ascend
> into heaven, I will exalt my throne above the stars
> of God: I will sit also upon the mount of the
> congregation, in the sides of the north: (13)

> I will ascend above the heights of the clouds; I
> will be like the most High (14) (Isaiah 14:12-14).

You will recall that under God's direction Solomon's
Temple had been erected upon Mount Moriah. And at the
time of dedication, the glory of God had filled this temple
with a cloud. It was here that Jehovah had put His name
and received worship as the one true God of Israel.

Actually it was to Israel alone that God had revealed Himself in a special way.

> We are thine: thou never barest rule over them;
> they were not called by thy name (Isaiah 63:19).

SATAN...THE GREAT IMITATOR

Since Satan is the great imitator of God . . . during the first
half of the Tribulation Period, or before, Satan permits
Israel to rebuild this temple that he might at this place and
in the temple erected to God, transfer worship from God
to himself.

And where Jehovah had put His name . . . Satan in turn
sets up his image and working through the False Prophet,
who directs worship to the Antichrist, leads the Jews astray
and fulfills that part of prophecy which was quoted before
as saying:

> I am come in my Father's name, and ye receive
> me not: if another shall come in his own name,
> him ye will receive (John 5:43).

So here we find many Jews welcoming and worshiping
Antichrist thinking that he is from God.

The sad fact is that the prophet of the Old Testament had prophesied of this day and Jesus, too had warned Israel, more than 1900 years ago, about this coming tribulation period.

Jeremiah spoke of this in the Old Testament, referring to it as the time of Jacob's trouble, when he said in Jeremiah 30:7:

> Alas! for that day is great, so that none is like it: it is even the time of Jacob's trouble, but he shall be saved out of it.

And we are fast approaching the day which Jeremiah, Isaiah, Daniel and the Lord Jesus and others had prophesied.

Now Satan will be fulfilling these prophecies exactly as they had been written. Antichrist will assume power and the temple will be erected. **And because Israel refuses to worship Satan as God, there will follow one of the greatest slaughters in history as Jacob's trouble begins.**

This shows the power of sin! God has given both the Jews and the Gentiles signs in the heaven and earth, but these are mocked by the people of this day. Is it no wonder that the Bible tells us:

> But as the days of Noah were, so shall also the coming of the Son of man be (Matthew 24:37).

The tragedy is that even under these new judgments which redouble with intensity, the world will still continue to worship Satan and not believe in the true God.

This will be the condition of the world at the close of the first 3½ years of the Tribulation Period.

What is now left for God to do when He is rejected of men?

The only thing left for Him to do is to follow His plan for the development of His kingdom during this closing period when there are false teachers and false preachers and people believing and worshipping a lie.

Therefore, He allows the second 3½ years of the Tribulation Period to occur in which this trial by fire awakens many thousands to accepting Christ as their personal Saviour and brings the Jew back to the fold into acknowledging Christ as Messiah, Saviour, Redeemer and Lord.

The Egyptians refer to Henry Kissinger as "The Magician." In 1973 he traveled 120,000 miles.

The Philadelphia Inquirer

This is one of the reasons why the second half of the Tribulation Period, commonly known as "Jacob's trouble," must come to pass.

SATAN'S ROLE IN
THE TRIBULATION PERIOD

During the first 3½ years Antichrist (the world ruler) and the False Prophet (the world church leader) have so fooled the world into believing that they are truly called of God and have truly brought peace to the earth . . . that now Satan can move into the next phase of his program and cause the people of the world to bow down and worship him.

To those who refuse, their refusal will heap on their heads terror and tragedy.

Jerusalem, the city of Peace, has been the scene of many bloody conflicts.

But God promised that the time would come when that city would be rebuilt and extended according to His blueprint. He also promised that after this the city would not be destroyed again.

We find this in Jeremiah 31:38-40:

> Behold, the days come, saith the Lord, that the city shall be built to the Lord from the tower of Hananeel unto the gate of the corner. (38)

> And the measuring line shall yet go forth over against it upon the hill Gareb, and shall compass about to Goath. (39)

> And the whole valley of the dead bodies, and of the ashes, and all the fields unto the brook of Kidron, unto the corner of the horse gate toward the east, shall be holy unto the Lord; it shall not be plucked up, nor thrown down any more for ever. (40)

As we previously stated, there will appear on the scene the Antichrist who will be head of the Federated States of Europe.

ANTICHRIST AND RUSSIA

In attempting to settle the Arab-Israeli dispute, he will side with Israel and back her claim to the land of Palestine against Russia.

Russia will back the Arabs' claim to Palestine (Ezekiel 38).

Because the Antichrist will make a pledge to protect Israel the Jews will no doubt flock back to Israel in unprecedented numbers.

The Scriptures seem to give us some indication that in this time Russia may part with her Jews and allow them to return to Israel. It is estimated that there are over 2 million Jews in Russia at present.

After this occurs, Russia, feeling she is all powerful, will probably make her move into the land of Israel.

God will allow this to happen because He will not tolerate His people looking to the Antichrist as their saviour. Therefore, the Jews will again be driven out of their land and many will flee from Israel and the two thirds of those left behind will be slain so that, alas, the soil of Israel will again be drenched with the blood of the children of Abraham.

> And it shall come to pass, that in all the land, saith the Lord, two parts therein shall be cut off and die; but the third shall be left therein (Zechariah 13:8).

> And among these nations shalt thou find no ease, neither shall the sole of thy foot have rest: but the Lord shall give thee there a trembling heart, and failing of eyes, and sorrow of mind: (65)

> And thy life shall hang in doubt before thee; and thou shalt fear day and night, and shalt have none assurance of thy life: (66)

> In the morning thou shalt say, Would God it were even! and at even thou shalt say, Would God it were morning! for the fear of thine heart wherewith thou shalt fear, and for the sight of thine eyes which thou shalt see (67) (Deuteronomy 28:65-67).

After this occurs may be the time when God will step in and devastate Russia and Russian Communism, including her allies as He has prophesied in Ezekiel 38:1-39:16.

It seems that this is the time that the Federated States of

Europe will move into this vacuum created by the defeat of Russia. It is at this time that Antichrist will rule over all the earth.

THE MARK OF THE BEAST (Antichrist)

In Revelation 13:15 we read that the False Prophet decrees "...that as many as would not worship the image of the beast (Antichrist) should be killed."

If you will look back at verse 7 of this same chapter you will read:

> And it was given unto him to make war with the saints, and to overcome them: and power was given him over all kindreds, and tongues, and nations.

It is then further revealed how the Antichrist will try to overcome the saints.

And this is how it will happen. He sets up this great religious system with himself (Antichrist) as its god. And in Revelation 13:16-17 we are told:

> And he causeth all, both small and great, rich and poor, free and bond, to receive a mark in their right hand, or in their foreheads: (16)
>
> And that no man might buy or sell, save he that had the mark, or the name of the beast, or the number of his name. (17)

Therefore, in that day it will be impossible to buy or sell without this identifying sign either on the back of your hand or on your forehead. When an individual refuses to submit to the authority of the Antichrist and will not allow this mark to be put on his body, he faces the consequences of either starving to death slowly or else being slain by a representative of the then existing government.

We already see the pattern being laid for this. The Social Security number is fast becoming the universal number in buying a car, in being admitted to a hospital, in securing a loan, etc. The privilege of buying gas on a certain day depends on whether you have an odd or an even number.

PEKING. — U.S. Secretary of State Henry Kissinger told Premier Chou En-lai and other Chinese leaders yesterday that "friendship with China is one constant factor of American foreign policy" in the future, no matter who is in the White House.

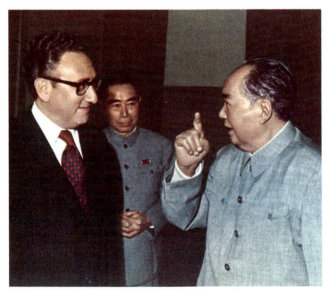

Henry Kissinger meets Chairman Mao, February 17, 1973 as Premier Chou En-lai looks on. A similar meeting took place again in China November 10-14, 1973.

WHAT IS THE IDENTIFYING MARK

What this identifying mark will be . . . the Lord has not desired to make clear to us at this time. Nor can we know at this time the identity of Antichrist.

It may be the number "**666**" which is the number of MAN and stops short of the perfect number 7. Thus "**666**" may well represent the humanistic and sinful counterfeit Satanic Trinity falling short of the divine 777, and catering to lost and fallen man. You will recall man was created on the *sixth* day, and in Daniel 3:1-7 we read where Nebuchadnezzar's image to be worshipped was sixty cubits in height, six cubits wide and six instruments of music summoned the worshippers to worship him.

Or, it may be that Antichrist's name or title may add up to a total equalling "**666**" using the following ancient number code (this code could be applied to any alphabetical language):

A = 1	F = 6	K = 20	P = 70	U = 300
B = 2	G = 7	L = 30	Q = 80	V = 400
C = 3	H = 8	M = 40	R = 90	W = 500
D = 4	I = 9	N = 50	S = 100	X = 600
E = 5	J = 10	O = 60	T = 200	Y = 700
				Z = 800

Those people who do carry this mark will most likely prefer to have it on the back of their right hand so that it can readily be seen in the act of signing checks and buying.

It is conceivable that the daily papers will contain a list of the names of those who have been killed the day before who have refused to have this mark imprinted on their forehead or on their hand. According to Revelation 20:4, the instrument of death would seem to be the guillotine, or some similar beheading agent.

With the reign of terror which demands that everyone wear the identifying mark of the Antichrist, and with plague judgments of the Lord, there will be a mass exodus in which the Jews will try to flee from this destruction into what to them will be unfamiliar and unfriendly territory.

Some Bible scholars believe the area they will flee to is the city of Petra. Others suggest a flight into the wilderness of the nations of the world.

WHO IS ANTICHRIST?

There have been many views expounded on exactly who Antichrist will be.

However, it is important to keep in mind that Antichrist will **not** be revealed until after the Rapture (When the saints rise to meet Christ in the air).

After the Christians are taken up from earth to meet Christ at the Rapture — then the person of Antichrist will be identified and revealed. According to 2 Thessalonians 2:4, the proof of his identity comes when he sits in the rebuilt Temple in Jerusalem and declares himself to be God.

The Bible does give us some key characteristics that will expose his true identify as Antichrist.

1. **He will be popular and worshipped!**
   ...the whole earth was amazed and followed after the beast [Antichrist] ...and they worshiped the beast... (Revelation 13:3,4).

2. **He will be fearless!**
   ...Who is like the beast [Antichrist], and who is able to wage war with him? (Revelation 13:4)

3. **He will persecute the Tribulation Saints!**
   And it was given to him to make war with the saints and to overcome them... (Revelation 13:7)

4. **He will be a world dictator!**
   ...authority over every tribe and people and tongue and nation was given to him (Revelation 13:7).

5. **He will be a maker of peace treaties!**
   And he will make a firm covenant [treaty] with the many for one week [one "seven" year period] with Israel (Daniel 9:27).

6. **He will not honor his peace treaty!**
   ...in the middle of the week [at 3½ years] he will put a stop to sacrifice...and on the wing of abominations will come one who makes desolate, even until a complete destruction...is poured out on the one who makes desolate (Daniel 9:27).

   He will break his pledge and stop the Jews from all their sacrifices, and as a climax to his terrible deeds, he will defile the sanctuary of God.

7. **He will have no respect for the religion of his race; nor will he embrace any religious conviction!**

   And he will show no regard for the gods of his fathers ...nor will he show regard for any other god; for he will magnify himself above them all (Daniel 11:37).

8. **He will change territorial boundaries!**

   ...he will give great honor to those who acknowledge him, and he will cause them to rule over many, and shall divide the land for gain (Daniel 11:39).

9. **He will be a skilled negotiator!**

   And at the latter end of their kingdom, when the transgressors [the apostate Jews] have reached the fullness [of their wickedness, exceeding the limits of God's mercy], a king of fierce countenance and understanding dark trickery and craftiness, shall stand up (Daniel 8:23).

10. **His armies will be destroyed and he will be cast alive into the Lake of Fire!**

    And the beast [Antichrist] was seized, and with him the false prophet who performed the signs in his presence, by which he deceived those who had received the mark of the beast [666] and those who worshiped his image; these two were thrown alive into the lake of fire which burns with brimstone. And the rest were killed with the sword... (Revelation 19:20,21).

There is some indication in Scripture that the Antichrist may be active on the world scene even before the Tribulation Period begins. This is based on 2 Thessalonians 2:3:

Don't be carried away and deceived regardless of what they say. For that day will not come until two things happen: first, there will be a time of great rebellion against God, and then the man of rebellion will come—the son of hell (The Living New Testament).

Then in verse 8 of the same chapter we read:

Then this wicked one will appear, whom the Lord Jesus will burn up with the breath of His mouth and destroy by His presence when He returns.

From this it would appear that the Antichrist may be known

THE JERUSALEM
POST

Price: ....

FRIDAY, NOVEMBER 30, 1975 ● KISLEV 5, 5734 ● ZIL-KI'ADA 6, 1393 ● VOL. XLIII, No. 13956

OPEN LETTER TO THE U.S. JEWISH PRESIDENTIAL MISSION:

DON'T REMAIN SILENT!
FIGHT KISSINGER'S PRESSURES!

In your visit here, you find a depressed people who overcame the great disadvantage of a surprise attack (remember Pearl Harbor!) and by terrible sacrifices achieved a military victory. But the people face with dread Kissinger's destructive programme for our future. Please heed our message, and pass it on to the American people and especially to U.S. Jewry.

1. The people of Israel do not believe our government when it says "there is no U.S. pressure." We know that ruthless Kissinger pressure denied us the completion of the military victory due any people subjected to a vicious sneak attack (remember Pearl Harbor!); that ruthless Kissinger pressure seeks to save the encircled Third Army which would some day fight us again; that ruthless Kissinger pressure plans to deprive us of minimum vital defence areas, making self-defence immeasureably more difficult, reducing us to complete dependence on the whims of any U.S. Secretary of State.

2. In Korea and Vietnam the U.S.A. spent over $1 trillion and suffered over 300,000 casualties. The Middle East is far more vital to U.S. interests. Egypt and Syria are basically expansionist. In the past (Yemen poison gas war, 1958 Marines in Lebanon, 1971 threat to Jordan) and inevitably in the future, they will clash with U.S. interests. We are saving U.S. Korea-Vietnam sacrifices. Appeasement of Arabs, like the appeasement of Hitler, is self-defeating. The faithful, complete Russian identification with the Arabs proves the so-called detente never truly existed. Instead, the U.S. is feeding and helping its greatest enemy to emasculate the U.S.A.'s most reliable ally in the Middle East.

3. The people of Israel are gravely concerned that our government has not appealed to U.S. Jewry to fight the terrible threat to Jewish and U.S. interest, but has done the opposite. We have not forgotten the Holocaust, the silence of Jewish leadership and the refusal to mobilize Jewry then.

4. Our hearts go out to Senator Jackson. We fully accept his ideas on the true U.S. interests here. We acclaim his support and his splendid struggle on behalf of Soviet Jewry. On the other hand, we are greatly ashamed and concerned over Kissinger's exploitation of his own supposed Jewish loyalties, as the means to lure us into his trap of appeasement.

5. The people of Israel desperately desire that the American people be made aware of the identity of American and Israeli interests, and that they accept Israel as a staunch ally — not as a servile puppet. As Jews and loyal Americans, your duty is to arouse America for the desperate fight against the Kissinger (Chamberlain) policy of appeasing aggressors.

Citizens for Prevention of a National Disaster

P.O.B. 36760, Tel Aviv.

to us (but not identifiable as Antichrist) before the Rapture occurs.

However, this is important. His real, diabolical, Satanic *character* is revealed only at the middle of the Tribulation, when he demands a type of worship which can only rightly be given unto God.

It is not God's purpose to reveal everything to us in this day and age.

(Some Bible scholars have even suggested that Antichrist, taking advantage of the unsettled conditions in the Middle East, will establish himself as the ruler of Iraq, the land upon which the ancient city of Babylon once stood.

In time he will attack and subdue three member states of the Mediterranean Confederacy which from then on will be ruled by Iraq as the center of this newly acquired empire.

This would make the prophetic "Babylon" of Revelation 17 and 18 literally Babylon Rebuilt. You will recall that Babylon was the center of the nations' first rebellion against God as recorded in the Tower of Babel episode in Genesis.)

What about his religion? Religiously, he will deny all authority but his own authority. He is called in Scriptures— The Lawless One.

The October, 1973 "Yom Kippur" War in the Middle East brought new problems to the world unleashing an avalanche of events that are drawing us even closer to the time of the Rapture.

The fourth Arab-Israeli war since the foundation of the Jewish state in 1948 spawned a host of perils. Not only did the combatants pay a fearsome price in blood and treasure but the conflict drew the United States and Russia into a near confrontation.

ENERGY CRISIS A PRELUDE

The United States torn between whether it should support the Arab nations or Israel . . . sided finally with Israel. Promptly the Arab nations stopped the flow of oil to the United States.

This sparked the famous November 7, 1973 Energy Crisis speech by President Richard Nixon. Gas stations were ordered closed on Sundays, a 55-mile per hour speed limit was enforced nationally.

"Spy on your Neighbor" programs began to rear their ugly head as some states suggested phoning a Complaint Center for those who waste energy.

Christmas tree lights were dimmed. Churches cancelled Christmas eve services. The nation and the world suddenly were caught in the mass hysteria of world trials . . . while a courier of peace, Henry Kissinger, flew furiously back and forth to China, to Russia and to Brussels and Geneva striving to restore peace.

These events are a prelude and a prototype of the chaos that will occur during the initial reign of Antichrist.

Time will certainly reveal the answers to these questions.

The important thing for the reader to know is not necessarily who Antichrist is but to recognize his need for the Saviour and to accept Jesus Christ as his personal Saviour and Lord.

If however, this is <u>not</u> done —you will recognize the Antichrist by the description we have given as to what he will do when he does come.

God alone can give genuine peace. Jesus is known as the Prince of Peace. Antichrist will try to take over this role and produce a so-called heaven on earth.

We will see the world become very enthusiastic about his reign and indeed some very marvelous things will be produced at that time. Great new cities may be built and science will no doubt make startling discoveries.

This will be an era in which man will be exalted to the skies but in Obadiah 1:4 the Lord promises:

> Though thou exalt thyself as the eagle, and though thou set thy nest among the stars, thence will I bring thee down, saith the Lord.

If you live during the reign of Antichrist . . . don't be fooled by his message of peace . . . for his main purpose is to bring a reign of death and destruction!

WHAT WILL YOU DO WITH JESUS?

After reading this book it should become evident to you that the world is **not** getting better and better.

What happens when it comes time for you to depart from this earth?

Then WHAT WILL YOU DO WITH JESUS?

Here are five basic observations in the Bible of which you should be aware:

1. ALL SIN — For all have sinned, and come short of the glory of God. (Romans 3:23)
2. ALL LOVED — For God so loved the world, that He gave His only begotten Son, that whosoever believeth in Him should not perish, but have everlasting life (John 3:16)
3. ALL RAISED — Marvel not at this: for the hour is coming, in which all that are in the graves shall hear his voice.

   And shall come forth; they that have done good, unto the resurrection of life; and they that have done evil, unto the resurrection of damnation. (John 5:28,29)
4. ALL JUDGED — ...we shall all stand before the judgment seat of Christ. (Romans 14:10)

   And I saw the dead, small and great, stand before God; and the books were opened...(Revelation 20:12)
5. ALL BOW — ...at the name of Jesus every knee should bow...(Philippians 2:10)

Right now, in simple faith, you can have the wonderful assurance of eternal life.

Ask yourself, honestly, the question....WHAT WILL I DO WITH JESUS?

God tells us the following:

   "...him that cometh to me I will in no wise cast out. (37) Verily, verily (truly) I say unto you, He that believeth on me (Christ) hath everlasting life" (47)—(John 6:37, 47).

He also is a righteous God and a God of indignation to those who reject Him....

   "...he that believeth not is condemned already, because he hath not believed in the name of the only begotten Son of God"—(John 3:18).

   "And whosoever was not found written in the book of life was cast into the lake of fire"—(Revelation 20:15).

YOUR MOST IMPORTANT DECISION IN LIFE

All of your riches here on earth—all of your financial security —all of your material wealth, your houses, your land will crumble into nothingness in a few years.

No matter how great your works—no matter how kind you are—no matter how philanthropic you are—it means nothing in the sight of God, because in the sight of God, your riches are as filthy rags.

"...all our righteousnesses are as filthy rags..." (Isaiah 64:6)

Christ expects you to come as you are, a sinner, recognizing your need of a Saviour, the Lord Jesus Christ.

Understanding this, why not bow your head right now and give this simple prayer of faith to the Lord.

My Personal Decision for CHRIST

"Lord Jesus, I know that I'm a sinner and that I cannot save myself by good works. I believe that you died for me and that you shed your blood for my sins. I believe that you rose again from the dead. And now I am receiving you as my personal Saviour, my Lord, my only hope of salvation. I know that I cannot save myself. Lord, be merciful to me, a sinner, and save me according to the promise of Your Word. I want Christ to come into my heart now to be my Saviour, Lord and Master."

Signed ....

Date ....

If you have signed the above, having just taken Christ as your personal Saviour and Lord...I would like to rejoice with you in your new found faith.

Write to me...Salem Kirban, Kent Road, Huntingdon Valley Penna. 19006...and I'll send you a little booklet to help you start living your new life in Christ.